Do You REALLY Want To Get Well?

Janis K. Johnson, MD

ISBN - 978-1-945773-00-6

Table of Contents

Forward

This book was originally written for those who are seriously ill, with cancer or some other chronic disease. However, I believe that any and everyone can use these simple, basic concepts, to achieve continuous vibrant health, if that is your goal.

What do I mean by vibrant health? Let's define it. Vibrant has two different meanings which both apply here.

> 1) Pulsating with vigor, vitality and energy

> 2) Produced as the result of vibration

A truly healthy body isn't just in a state of being "free from detectable disease". These days, with our increasingly toxic environment and stress-promoting culture, it is difficult to find someone who radiates vigor, vitality and energy. I can tell you that it is a goal worth pursuing and I challenge you to do the right things, long enough, so that you experience that feeling yourself.

What about the second definition: produced as the result of vibration? Not only your body, but every cell, every molecule within every cell, all the way down to its subatomic particles, have a vibration. These vibrations must be in alignment and in harmony if you want vibrant health. But how? It sounds impossible, a lot like trying to herd cats or chickens.

The good news is that you don't have to concern yourself with the complexity of managing all those trillions of particles and quintillion details. There are simple, doable ways to get it all moving harmoniously in the right direction. That is the road to vibrant health.

Vibrant health is a journey, not a destination. Just when you feel you've arrived, something changes and you need to adjust again. I know some of you are thinking, "what you're describing seems way out of reach, I just want to feel better and not die!" All I can say is, get on the path and see where it takes you. Many people start this journey and then jump off the path, back into their old destructive habits as soon as they start feeling better. The bottom line is - ***it's your choice***. The way you choose to live your life is up to you.

I hope you like adventures that take you to places where you've never been before. I encourage you to approach this as an adventure. And may you never be the same.

Introduction

I can assume that your health isn't as good as you would like it to be, or you wouldn't be reading this book. Unless, of course, you are reading it to find information to help someone you care about. If you have a serious or life-threatening illness, you may be feeling desperate to find an answer, any answer, to improve your situation.

In this short book I offer you an effective and practical approach anyone can use to turn their health around. Although it's simple, it isn't always easy. This book is for anyone who feels their health is sub-optimal and has a true desire to do something about it.

But why should you listen to me? Especially when much of my approach isn't very popular with mainstream, conventional medicine. The MD behind my name isn't a good enough reason. My medical education included exactly two hours of lectures on nutrition and a heavy emphasis on prescribing drugs to cover up symptoms. Conventional medical schools teach "sick care", not health care.

I suggest that you listen to someone who has what you want, that is, vibrant health, and has been where you are. So I'll give you a brief synopsis of my journey from life-threatening illness to vibrant health. You can find the full story in my biography, *Life Uncommon.*

By the age of thirty six, my body was what many doctors would call a "train wreck". It started with a near-fatal hang-gliding accident at the age of seventeen, followed by Myasthenia Gravis at the age of twenty six and Chronic Active Hepatitis B at age twenty seven. I was given a 5% chance of survival.

I am writing this book just after my 59th birthday. I don't use glasses - not even for reading. My blood pressure is like a ten year old and my blood sugar and weight are normal. In fact, all of my lab results are in the normal range and I take no medications. I haven't had a cold or flu in over 20 years. I have more energy than most people, despite some old damage. I enjoy vibrant health today.

I'm not the only person who is living proof that wellness is possible for anyone who is willing to do what it takes. Far from it. You probably know someone who has overcome a serious illness. So don't put your attention on statistics - they only apply to groups, not individuals. The uncommon person is just the common one, who has changed his thinking and habits.

This book isn't just for those in desperate situations, but to show anyone how to improve their health, energy and enjoyment of life. And that is what you can expect to get from consistently applying the ideas in this book. It is not meant to replace competent medical evaluation and treatment, but to give you control of your health and medical care - maybe for the first time in your life.

This book is intentionally short and not technical. It is meant to be re-read often, as the lifestyle changes described may take some time to implement. Your viewpoint and awareness will also change as you implement the ideas in this book. For those of you who would like to read more, you can find a list of interesting books in the Appendix. Many of those books will give you more details of the research and theory behind the conclusions I've drawn and applied to date to achieve excellent health.

I encourage you to start your journey to vibrant health today. Don't be the person who waits until it's too late and misses their opportunity. Be the person that other people call a walking miracle - so full of life and love, that instead of pitying you, they can't help but feel inspired.

All you have to do is to keep reading, then apply what you learn. You **can** take control of your health and life. Start now!

Chapter 1 - The First Step

**"The journey of a thousand miles
begins with one step."**

Lao Tzu

How teachable are you? What exactly do I mean? Let's explore that in two parts: How willing are you to learn? How willing are you to accept change?

Since you are still reading this book, I will assume that you feel there may be something for you to learn here and you have the willingness to learn it. Good. If not, please only read this book when you are feeling that willingness to learn. Otherwise, you are wasting your time.

It is your thoughts and decisions that have brought you to this exact point in your life where you find yourself right now. This is the time to become real honest with yourself - no one else, just yourself. Start by becoming aware and noticing what makes your body better, or worse. We'll discuss this more.

I'm telling you up front that to change your health and well being, you will have to change some things in your life. Well, duh! Continuing to do the same things and expecting a different result isn't sane or logical. Yes, it's true that we all have reasons for being sick, but without changing those things, you won't get well ... at least not for long. You are not going to get positive results from inappropriate thoughts, choices and actions. This may not be what you want to hear, but it's the truth.

Let's say you want to improve your tennis game. You search and find a tennis coach who consistently gets excellent results with his students. It would be stupid to take instruction from someone who doesn't have a high rate of success. It would be equally silly to ignore that successful coach and keep swinging your racquet the same way, lesson after lesson, never improving your game. Don't you agree?

How willing are you to accept change? What are you willing to give up in order to have vibrant health? Do you have an "I'll do whatever it takes" attitude, or an "I just couldn't do that" kind of attitude? As you go through this book, become aware of how teachable you are by noticing how willing you are to accept the changes suggested here. Do you quickly find excuses for not changing? How willing are you to give up some bad habits? Those same habits that have eroded your health over the years and adopt some new habits that you've thus far avoided? Any particular habits come to mind?

For some of us, we wait until it's a matter of life and death before we are ready to make those needed changes. Hopefully, you haven't waited that long, and can make these changes gradually, over several months. But if you have, you may need to make more and faster changes to turn your situation around. Everyone is unique, with different circumstances. This is something you will have to figure out as you go.

So now, it's time to step up to the plate and take responsibility for your health. It's not your doctor's responsibility. It's not your partner's, not your family's – it's yours. It's **your** body and **your** life. You know your situation and body better than anyone, and only you can make those decisions, after you have the information you need. You may be unsure how to answer some of these questions. Just give it your best shot and in time, you will discover the answers you need.

What information do I need to learn to improve my health?

_____

_____

_____

_____

_____

How am I going to get that information?

_____

_____

_____

_____

Which habits do I already know I need to change and why?

_____

_____

_____

_____

_____

_____

How much time am I willing to spend each week on the activities that I've decided I need to do?

_____

_____

_____

How much money am I willing to spend to get well/healthier?

_____

_____

_____

I encourage you to re-read this short chapter every week and answer the questions again, in detail, each week, as the answers will change as you gain more knowledge and experience.

Now, I'm going to tell you something that you may find unbelievable.

Chapter 2 - What? Are You Kidding?

"I thank God for my handicaps, for through them, I have found myself, my work and my God."

Helen Keller

Your illness or injury is a great gift. It is an invitation to begin a voyage of self discovery and personal growth. You may have already received many such invitations in the past. Most of you didn't even RSVP, much less accept the invitation.

How do I know this? My own experience has taught me that if we don't pay attention to both our thoughts and our body's signals and responses, we'll get another chance. The disturbances just get bigger, uglier and more serious until we finally say, "OK, OK, I get it! I need to make different and better choices."

Only some of us still don't get it, and keep paying, again and again, for our lack of awareness.

Think about the last time you went on a junk food, sugar or drinking binge. Or a binge of self-pity, holding onto anger, or worrying about things you imagined could go "wrong"? How much time and energy did you put into justifying and explaining why you did it? I bet you didn't spend a whole lot of time being thankful for the wake up call, while you were feeling bad. That's because it's impossible to feel bad and be grateful at the same time.

If you are reading this, it is very likely that you are overweight. Why do I say that? Because people who are overweight have a greater risk of heart disease, stroke, cancer, diabetes, arthritis, gallbladder disease, autoimmune disorders and breathing problems. How often do you explain your condition, to yourself or others, as "bad genes" or some other explanation beyond your control? Who do *you* blame?

So now you have a serious illness. You've gotten the BIG WAKE UP CALL. The good news is that there is almost no condition that can't be reversed, as long as you are willing to do the right things, consistently, long enough. And for you, long enough just might be for the rest of your life.

"But," you say, "what about _____?" (you fill in the blank with the name of a person who had horrible health habits and seemed to get away with it) Obviously, you're not that person. So let's not waste time with this line of thought. It not only won't help you achieve vibrant health, it is actually detrimental. You'll see why when we get to work in Chapter 4.

Right now, let's get started with a little adjustment in perspective. This exercise may bring up all sorts of interesting thoughts and emotions. If not, you need to keep doing it until you do get in touch with some of these. Your voyage of self discovery begins now.

With a pen and paper (or use the space provided on the next page), write down all the reasons you are thankful and grateful for your illness or injury. No, I'm not kidding. You don't need to show this to anyone else; just be completely honest with yourself. You are the one person you don't ever want to lie to.

You may realize that it has allowed you to get out of some tasks or situations that have made you feel trapped or overwhelmed. (Won't be going back to that job, hee hee!) Or, it may seem like a way of taking revenge on someone who you feel has wronged or neglected you. (Now, they'll be sorry) Being sick or injured may be a way for you to get the attention you've wanted and haven't gotten in the past. Even if it seems weird, whatever comes to mind, write it down.

Often, we aren't even aware of the emotions we suppress in order to be "socially acceptable"- but suppressing these emotions can destroy our health. You may feel blame, guilt, grief, hopelessness, fear or anger as you do this. There is no wrong answer or wrong emotion.

You may have trouble staying with the idea of being thankful and think about how unfair it all is. Just put it all down on paper, with today's date. Keep answering the question, "Why am I thankful and grateful for my condition?" until you run out of answers or have a realization. You may just discover why you got this disease/health problem in the first place. Use the rest of this page or write in your own journal.

Now, we're ready to get down to business.

Chapter 3 – Back To the Basics

"Natural forces within us are the true healers of disease."

Hippocrates

Let's get back to the basics, all the way back to Hippocrates, who has been called the Father of Western Medicine. Most of us are familiar with his two most famous quotes: **"Let food be thy medicine and medicine be thy food"** and **"First, do no harm."** Actually, there's a bit more to that last quote: **"As to diseases, make a habit of two things — to help, or at least, to do no harm."**

So, how can I help you in a way that will at least do no harm? I will give you the benefit of my education, observations and experience, so that you are in a better position to take control of your own health and life. Feel free to reject or disagree with anything I say. You must prove for yourself what is true for you.

Before going on, there are a few lesser-known quotes of Hippocrates that I'd like to share with you:

"The natural healing force within each of us is the greatest force in getting well."

With that said, this is what I have come to believe: The body is a self-balancing, self-healing system. No doctor ever healed anyone. Your body has what it needs to regain that balanced state which I call health. Your job is to give it the exercise and raw materials it needs to work with, and not sabotage it, by filling it with things that interfere with its natural potential to heal.

Let's say you own a factory. To produce products in sufficient volume to be a viable business, you have to supply it with all the raw materials and skilled labor it needs. You have to clean and maintain the machines properly and carefully train the workers who operate them, so that those machines aren't damaged by misuse. If you use the wrong fuel, for example, putting gasoline in a diesel engine, the machine will not run well and may be totally ruined. Give that machine excess oil or electricity, and again, you may totally ruin it. When one or two machines aren't working well, they hold up the whole line. Do you see how that could be?

Every one of your approximately 37 trillion cells is like a tiny factory, which makes specialized products to support the entire community, which is your body. Some of those products are more vital than others. If enough of those cells fail to make their products, or make poor-quality products, the whole group's survival is lessened and your body is less healthy, if not outright sick. When enough of those miniature factories stop working, or start turning out sub-standard or destructive products, you will have an identifiable, label-able disease to discuss with your friends and family.

This brings us to another quote from Hippocrates:

"It is far more important to know what person the disease has, than what disease the person has."

I remember in my residency how patients were referred to as "the chronic bronchitis in room 514", or "the colon cancer in 305". The point here is that we are all unique; two people with the same disease may have a very different expression of that disease and may need different approaches to healing.

We are not walking physical maladies, who just need a correct diagnosis, surgery and drugs to patch us up. The underlying cause must be found and addressed, otherwise the same, or maybe a different system will break down before long.

The body by itself is a complex association of systems that seeks to survive in the moment and can make rapid changes in order to accomplish just that. It doesn't have the same success in long-term planning. For example, when you feel anger or fear, your blood pressure increases and your blood flow patterns change, directing blood to the brain, heart and muscles, and away from the skin, so that you're ready for a fight or a quick getaway. Most of these responses are automatic, controlled by the autonomic nervous system. We don't have a lot to say about that, but we can control, in large part, what we feed our minds and bodies.

When one is in a state of chronic fear, anxiety, anger or resentment, the body's solution, which is great for immediate survival in a dangerous situation, doesn't work so well long term. It's destructive, causing cardiovascular disease, disturbances of digestion and metabolism, malfunction of the immune system and cancer. Our choices are to either moderate the stressful influences of our environment, or speed down the path of illness and physical breakdown. That is our point of control. What do we feed our bodies and minds? How do we use our bodies and minds?

One last quote from Hippocrates:

"That which is used - develops. That which is not used wastes away."

This applies to both the body and the mind. Even if you are bedridden, move your body to whatever extent that you can. Most people can walk for 15 minutes a day - even if it's three five minute walks to start. You can also exercise your mind in a way that contributes to health! How much time do you spend learning new things? How much time do you spend everyday being thankful and grateful for all that you have and can do. And you can stop indulging in destructive thought patterns (blame, resentment, self pity, helplessness); if not used, they too will waste away.

Now for this chapter's exercise!

Write down as many things as you can that you could be doing to better your health, but aren't doing, keeping the capabilities and resources that you already have in mind.

Now choose ONE, just one, that you are willing to do, and DO that!

(It's a good idea to keep a journal, so that months from now you can reflect on the changes you made. It will help you determine which changes moved you in the right direction and which didn't work as well for you.)

Chapter 4 - The Most Important Thing

"The fact that the mind rules the body is, in spite of the neglect of biology and medicine, the most fundamental fact which we know about the process of life."

--Franz Alexander, M.D.

If you were only willing to change one thing, just one, what would be the most important thing? What you eat or don't eat? Exercise? Type of medical treatment? Your environment? Your relationships?

No, it's your thoughts.

You are probably thinking, "Oh no, I didn't think it would be this hard! You want me to change the way of thinking that is comfortable and familiar to me? How can I do that?!"

Don't stress about it; there is an approach that makes it easier. It will still require some awareness and discipline on your part, and because it's **your** mind, no one else can do this for you.

So before you throw this book across the room and scream, "That's impossible! I think thousands of thoughts every day. I can't do that!". Please consider this:

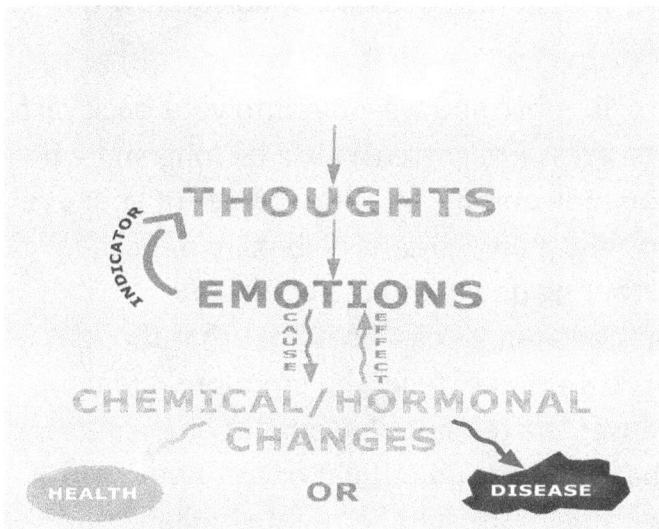

You and only you create your thoughts. You may allow others or your environment to **influence** your thoughts, but you have the final word. Your thoughts **cause** your emotions. In turn, your emotions cause chemical and hormonal changes in your body. And those chemicals that are released do have an effect on your emotions. You may not control the way your body responds to your emotions, that is basically automatic, but you can affect which emotions you cause your body to experience. The way your body reacts to those chemical signals determines the state of your health. Let's take a look at how this works.

Suppose you walk out into your back yard. The grass has gotten a little bit long and when you look quickly, from the corner of your eye, you see a dark green coil behind a rock slithering down into the grass. You immediately think, "SNAKE!!" That thought makes you feel fear. The emotion of fear causes the release of a long list of chemicals that prepare you to fight or run away. You become more alert, your pupils dilate, your heart rate and blood pressure increase, digestion grinds to a halt. The body experiences "stress". This isn't a problem in the short term. In fact, it's very necessary for survival that the body is able to quickly respond to potentially dangerous situations.

When you realize that what you saw was just part of the garden hose and not a snake, you will still feel afraid for a while because those "stress" response chemicals are still circulating in your body, prolonging the emotion that caused them to be released in the first place. As those chemicals are deactivated and cleared out, the feeling of fear and stress goes away and the body returns to its normal balance. Unless...

If the body is constantly being bombarded with negative emotions, those stress chemicals remain active, affecting every cell and every organ in your body. The weakest link will break first.

That is your warning that there is something you are doing that you *shouldn't* be doing, or that there is something you *should* be doing that you aren't. Make sense? More about this later.

Looking at the diagram, you can see there are several points at which the chemical/hormonal balance of your body can be affected. Western medicine attempts to alter these chemicals directly, by means of drugs. How well do you think that will work, in the long-term, if YOU keep bombarding the cells of your body with the same thoughts and emotions that created the problem in the first place?

What exactly do I mean by negative emotion? It's simple. It's a response that feels bad to you, because it produces an unwanted sensation or state of mind. This could include emotions like apathy, grief, despair, hopelessness, blame, shame, regret, exasperation, hate, anger, pity, or boredom, just to name a few. So obviously, a positive emotion is one that makes you feel good, or at least better; like enthusiasm, appreciation, hopefulness, certainty, compassion, peacefulness, contentment, excitement, love, cheerfulness, joy!

Now, take out your pen or pencil again and write down every example of a negative emotion and a positive emotion that you can think of in the space below. Feel free to add to the list later if you think of more. Use words in describing those feelings that are most meaningful to you.

<u>Negative Emotion</u> (Feels Bad)

<u>Positive Emotions</u> (Feels Good)

Chapter 4 - The Most Important Thing

Which things, people and situations do you let influence you to feel more negative than positive emotions? Write down those things, people, and situations that seem to elicit positive emotions.

<u>Negative Influences</u> <u>Positive Influences</u>

Chapter 4 - The Most Important Thing

Alright, so have you figured out how to be aware when you are thinking negatively - without having to monitor every thought? That's right! It's your emotions. They are your indicators of what you are thinking. It is impossible to feel good when your thoughts are focused on what makes you feel bad, and it is equally impossible to feel bad when you are thinking about people, things and situations that are positive, loving and supportive.

A Word About Your Emotional Environment

When I talk about emotional environment, this includes the objects, plants, animals and people that live with and around you. Who and what do you allow in your space? Is your home environment safe and nurturing? Which pets, plants, things and people elicit positive emotions and which do you feel are more of a piss off than a pay off? It's time to take a good long, honest look at the influences you have decided to allow in your environment and change those that are leading you down the wrong path. Sometimes it's necessary to get out of our usual environment, so that we can see it more objectively, and turn our situation around.

Take a walk through your house. Do you find yourself being drawn to some rooms and others repel you? Are there cluttered areas that you don't even want to look at? Maybe it's time to throw out those things that clearly don't contribute to your happiness. Now, look in your closet. Do you wear certain clothes because someone has told you to dress that way, or do you dress in a way that makes *you* feel good? When you really want to get well, you will take steps to create the most comfortable, loving and uplifting environment that you can. If not now, then when?

If you had a "friend" who brought a big, stinking bag of garbage over to your house, every time they came to visit, and dumped it in the middle of your living room - infesting your home with cockroaches and rats, would you keep inviting them over? Would they still be your friend if they did that? What would you do if they promised not to do it anymore

- 37 -

and then brought more garbage the next time they came over? So why would you let anyone, especially those who claim to love and care about you, fill your mind with negative "thought garbage" that undermines your health and happiness?

It comes down to two choices, handle them so that they stop doing that, or disconnect from their influence. This is easier to do with a neighbor or casual acquaintance than with a family member or close friend. There are two free courses called "The Cause of Suppression" and 'Solutions for a Dangerous Environment" to help you handle these kind of situations. You can find them online at http://www.scientology.org/courses.html I am not promoting any religion or philosophy, only sharing with you what I have found that worked and still works for me, because I haven't gotten sick in over 20 years.

Next, would you let a stranger come into your home every night, tell you all the bad news they had been able to find, and encourage you and your family to engage in behaviors that will destroy your health and happiness? Of course not! Then why are you still watching TV or reading the newspaper?! You have control over what you choose to read and watch. Be at least as careful about how you feed your mind as you are about how you feed your body. If you don't understand why I say this, go back and look at the diagram at the beginning of this chapter again.

By now you've probably had some ideas about what things and people in your life are contributing more to your illness than to your happiness. So here's one last list for this chapter:

Things I need to change and people I need to handle in my current environment:

Do You REALLY Want To Get Well?

Don't worry about *how* you are going to do this right now. Just make the decision NOW to change these things. If you are unsure about a particular person, I suggest you do the free online courses and keep reading; it will become clear to you.

We've already talked about changing things in your life; that is, if you want your life and health to improve. So, now let's talk about the way you take care of your body, if you REALLY want to get well.

Chapter 5 - Nutrition

"If we could give every individual the right amount of nourishment and exercise, not too little and not too much, we would have found the safest way to health."

Hippocrates

First, let's look at "nutrition" in a different way. We could say it is the process by which living organisms obtain food and use it for growth, metabolism, and repair. But let's look a little further at the definition of the word "nourish".

Nourish: To supply with what is necessary for life, health, and growth; to strengthen and build up. This is a bit different approach to nutrition. To nourish the body is to give it what is needed to strengthen and build it up, while avoiding those things that either tear it down, or just don't contribute to health.

So let's stop thinking of food in terms of entertainment, that is, eating something just because it tastes good or makes you feel better temporarily.

Excellent nutrition is possible, even in this day and age of depleted farmland and chemical-loving agribusiness. If you will take the time to learn how to get it.

For simplicity, I divide those things that are typically eaten in the Western world into three categories: Food, Toxic Food, and Non-Food.

<u>Foods</u>

Organically grown fruits & veggies
Raw organic honey, stevia, lucuma
Fish harvested from clean waters
Raw, whole, organic dairy
Foods dehydrated at 105F or less
Organic free-range meat, poultry, eggs
Himalayan pink salt, Celtic salt or clean sea salt
Organic herbs

Organic seeds, nuts, beans
Organic, mechanically cold-pressed oils
Non-GMO organic grains and grasses

Toxic Foods

Conventionally-grown or GMO produce
All GMO or refined & processed sugars
Farmed fish/fish raised in polluted waters
Conventional, pasteurized or homogenized
dairy products
Most processed or packaged foods
Conventionally raised meat, poultry and eggs
Table salt (some contain fluoride)
 Non-organic, chemically decaffeinated or
flavored coffees, teas, drinks, herbs
Conventional seeds, nuts, beans
Conventional heat or chemically extracted oils,
canola oil (Rapeseed)
Conventional/GMO grains and grasses

Non-Foods

Pesticides, herbicides, fungicides
Artificial sweeteners

Food dyes
Hormones
Drugs
Chemical additives
Antibiotics
Steroids
"Spices" that are really chemicals (MSG)
Flavor enhancers (MSG)
Artificial flavors
Artificial fats
Preservatives
Corn starch
High fructose corn syrup
Alcohol

This table is not comprehensive, just a general guideline. Yes, some herbs and organically grown produce may still contain contaminants like lead, arsenic or fluoride, if those are in the air or soil where they are grown. And some conventionally-grown produce may be fairly clean. It is up to you to find good sources for your food. Yes, the information on labels can be misleading or incomplete. The goal here is to increase your awareness, and then do the best you can. The body can tolerate and eliminate small amounts of some toxins quite well, *if* it is given the nourishment it needs. Don't think in terms of "giving up" foods you enjoy. Instead crowd out those "foods" containing toxins and poisons with cleaner, more nutrient-dense alternatives.

Here are the latest lists I could find of the Dirty Dozen (12 most contaminated conventionally grown fruits and veggies, listed in order of contamination) and the Clean 15 (cleanest conventionally grown)

Dirty Dozen   # Clean 15

Dirty Dozen	Clean 15
1. Strawberries	1. Avocados
2. Apples	2. Corn (non-GMO)
3. Nectarines	3. Pineapples
4. Peaches	4. Cabbage
5. Celery	5. Sweet Peas
6. Grapes	6. Onions
7. Cherries	7. Asparagus
8. Spinach	8. Mangos
9. Tomatoes	9. Papayas
10. Bell Peppers	10. Kiwi
11. Cherry Tomatoes	11. Eggplant
12. Cucumbers	12. Honeydew
	13. Grapefruit
	14. Cantaloupe
	15. Cauliflower

Do you really need me to tell you that you should probably be drinking more pure water, eating more organic fruits and vegetables and less processed, chemical-laden foods? What 2 or 3 changes can you think of that you KNOW make you feel better, more energetic, mentally clearer and happier?

If you expected me to give you a 7 or 30 day diet plan, recommend specific supplements, spelling out exactly what you should eat and when, I apologize for disappointing you. There are over 100 different dietary theories and each one is right for someone. There is no one-size-fits-all plan. You are an individual. Only you can determine what is best for your body, at any given time. You'll know by the way you feel. But you may have to follow your new nutrition plan for one to six weeks, or more, before you are sure.

And you may go through some rough times, commonly called a "Detox reaction" if you change your eating pattern dramatically. Consider for a moment how many years you chose an unhealthy diet and lifestyle before you became really ill. If you try to fix it in a week, or a month, you are going to be quite uncomfortable, which won't help you continue those new habits.

If you continue eating foods that you are allergic or sensitive to, you won't feel good and it may confuse you. Unfortunately, conventional scratch testing or RAST tests for food allergies aren't very reliable, economical or convenient. Food sensitivities change over time; some go away while new ones can appear. You need a way to determine which foods your body is saying "NO!" to.

Here is a simple test you can do yourself, to identify those foods that your body reacts to badly. It is called the Pulse Test. If you can count to 100, you can do it. It was developed and used in the 1950's by Dr. Arthur F. Coca, MD, with astonishing results. The book is now in the public domain (free) and can be found online at http://soilandhealth.org/wpcontent/uploads/02/0201hyglibcat/020108.coca.pdf.

I encourage you to take the time to read it. Here are the basics, taken directly from his book, so you can get started right away:

"On the day the test is started, each "meal" may be limited to a single, simple food. The pulse is counted in the morning before rising and again just before the first meal.

Thirty minutes after the meal the pulse is counted, and again at sixty minutes after the meal.

Immediately after the 60 minute count, another single food is eaten, and again the pulse-count is taken after the two half-hour intervals; and so on through the day. A record is kept of the foods eaten and of the pulse-counts.

The injurious foods are recognized by the abnormal speed-up of the pulse. *(10 or more beats/minute increase)** When these foods are dropped from the diet the allergic symptoms often disappear as if by magic.

That, in essence, is the procedure."

explained later in his book

Another method to determine which foods are best for you is kinesiology, or muscle testing, which you can learn to do on yourself. (see Appendix)

After many years of personal research, much of which was contradictory and confusing, I have concluded that the optimum approach to nutrition *for me,* is a cross between Dr. Terry Wahls' Diet and the approach described in "The China Study," which is a 27 year study of the effect of nutrition patterns on various diseases. I drew this conclusion only after trying it myself and finding that I felt better, had less pain and had the blood pressure and lab results of a healthy 20 year old, when I ate this way.

I eat 15-20 servings of fresh fruits and vegetables daily, about 80% of it raw. That includes 3 cups of green leafy vegetables, 3 cups of high sulfur (garlic, onions, cabbage family*) vegetables and 3 cups of highly colored fruits and veggies. Some is in the form of juice (8-16 oz daily) and some as whole food. I take a digestive enzyme capsule when I eat cooked food. In addition, I eat 2 Brazil nuts daily (for selenium), 1-2 T of coconut oil, 1 T of olive oil and 1-2 cloves of garlic daily.

I get more than enough protein (10-15% of my daily calories) without eating any animal protein, but will occasionally use raw goat milk, organic free-range eggs from my own chickens, and an ounce or two of fish or organic grass-fed beef. I eat beans/legumes once or twice a week. I aim for 10-15% protein (no more than half from animal sources), 15-20% fat, 65-70% carbohydrate from fruits and vegetables (no refined sugars or grain). I use various supplements when I travel. Bear in mind, this is what I do to stay healthy, after damage to my joints, nervous system, thyroid, kidneys and liver. If I was ill, this basic plan might be quite different.

*Cabbage family (or Brassicas) includes cabbage, bok choy, rapini, Brussels sprouts, broccoli, cauliflower, broccoflower (Romanesco), kale, mustard greens, collard greens, kohlrabi, turnips and rutabaga.

Chapter 6 - Moving Your Body

What most people would call "exercise" can be so unpleasant, inconvenient and expensive that very few actually do it. There is an easier way. Like with nutrition, we first need to change the way we think about moving our bodies.

Bodies lose strength and flexibility quickly if we stop moving. Immobilize a limb in a cast for six weeks, the muscles atrophy and the joint(s) get(s) stiff. Restoring normal strength and range of motion can be uncomfortable and time consuming.

A sedentary lifestyle contributes to many unhealthy conditions and outright disease; obesity, diabetes, heart disease, arthritis and cancer - just to name a few. Without getting too technical, this is what happens when we sit on our butts, or lie around in bed most of the day. We take shallow breaths, delivering less oxygen to all our tissues. This decreases our metabolic rate and effects many biochemical pathways, causing more acid to build up in cells and starting the downward spiral into cellular dysfunction, aging and eventual disease.

Start by making some simple changes. Take the stairs instead of the elevator. Park far away from the door and walk for a few minutes when you shop, go to work or appointments. It adds up, and will also save you a lot of dings in your car doors. If your work requires long hours of sitting, get up every hour or two, stretch, breathe deeply and walk around for a few minutes. You'll actually get more done. Make housework an aerobic activity; do it quickly, with energy, so that you work up a sweat.

The following list of activities are suggestions that you can try, until you find the moves that are right for you. Remember, you don't have to be able to do them perfectly. There is tremendous benefit in just making the attempt. If you persist, you will eventually build up the strength and endurance to master them. They can all be done at home. They require no or minimal equipment and can be modified if you currently have limitations.

1. Walking

Yes, just plain old unhurried walking to start, gradually increasing your speed until you can walk a mile in 15 minutes, or 4 miles in an hour. Outdoors is best, breathing fresh, clean air. Bring your dog along for company.

2. Rebounding
(Bouncing on a mini-trampoline)

You can get a rebounder on Amazon.com for about $40. The benefits of rebounding include cardiovascular conditioning, increased venous return and lymph flow (detoxification), improved posture and balance, and strengthening the immune system. Start by gently bouncing, without your feet leaving the surface for a few minutes and increase as your endurance improves. When you can do 15 minutes comfortably, then try walking, jogging or doing other exercises while bouncing on the rebounder. Use a stabilizing bar if you have balance issues. Put on your favorite music and enjoy!

3. The Five Tibetan Rites
(http://www.t5t.com/5-Tibetans-Free-Downloads)

Start by doing (or attempting to do) one to three repetitions of each, in order. Be aware of the feedback your body is giving you as you gradually increase the number of repetitions. It isn't a race. You will benefit even if you never reach the full 21 repetitions, 2-3 times per day. These movements are for restoring and balancing energy, not for strength, although they do increase both flexibility and strength. Many find that spending just ten minutes per day doing the Five Tibetans increases their energy, mental clarity and focus, while it reduces stress.

4. Pilates

This is a form of exercise developed by Joseph Pilates in the 1920's to strengthen the core muscles and correct muscle imbalances while improving posture and flexibility. Pilates exercises don't emphasize doing a lot of repetitions for each move, but instead, doing each exercise fully and precisely, giving you significant results in a shorter time than you would imagine. This can be done at home without a ball, bands or even a mat. I learned from a video, which you can check out at your local library. Or you can go to a class. Many find their joint and back pain decreases or completely goes away after a week or two.

5. Qi Gong or Tai Chi

Learning to control your life force energy through Qi Gong promotes healing by getting stuck energy flowing, relieves stress and teaches you how to breathe, while improving strength and balance. You can get instructional videos (I like Lee Holden's Modern Qi Gong course), or take a class to learn this.

I'm sure there are many other approaches to getting the body moving. Many of my friends swear by Hatha Yoga. The five I list here are just the ones that have given me good results personally. I encourage you to do whatever activities you enjoy. Dance! Garden! Ride a bicycle! Hike a nature path! Just get moving!

A word about breathing. Most people take little, shallow breaths most of the day and night. Any exercise that is vigorous enough to get you taking deep breaths will increase oxygenation and benefit every (normal) cell in your body. Remind yourself to take some deep, calming breaths often throughout your day. Cancerous cells, the organism that causes tuberculosis and abnormal cells that create lots of acid anaerobically won't like that extra oxygen. Oh, too bad.

I am often asked what a typical day for me looks like, so here it is:

8-12 oz of water, sometimes with lemon, soon after I get up, usually between 5am and 6am.

Read/study for 30 minutes.

Take a 20-30 minute walk outside (regardless of the weather).

Do the Five Tibetans or Qi Gong.

Drink a cup of weak coffee with 1 teaspoon of honey and 1 T coconut oil or raw organic goat milk about 7am.

Work for 2 hours.

Take a break and rebound for 10-15 minutes.

Drink 8-12 oz of fresh juice at about 9:30am (mostly veggies with ½ of a green apple) This gives me 7-8 servings of fresh, raw fruits and veggies, including barley or wheat grass. Followed by 12-16 oz of alkaline water. (If I get hungry before lunch, I eat a piece of fruit.)

Work for 2 hours.

Substantial lunch around noon to 1pm, with both raw and cooked veggies (fresh from my garden, as much as possible). 1-2T of organic cold-pressed oil. I don't usually eat grains (especially no corn and wheat, since so much of it is GMO).

Work for 2-3 hours.

Afternoon break at 3-4pm, a snack of fruit and 2 Brazil nuts or I just walk through my garden and nibble on whatever is ready to pick. Drink 8-16 oz of water or tea made from lemon grass, ginger or other things I grow myself. By now, I've eaten about 80% of my food for the day.

Work for 2 more hours.

Light dinner no later than 6pm, usually salad, soup or leftover food from lunch.

Study and spend time with my husband/friends in the evening.

I shower with non-toxic products (soap and shampoo) that I make myself.

I may do more Qi Gong, the 5 Tibetans again, or another 10 minutes of rebounding in the evening, if I'm at home or have access to a rebounder.

Again, this is a routine that works for me. I'm not suggesting that it is right for everyone. You will have to find what works for you, your schedule and your life.

Chapter 7 - Environmental Factors

"When we know our beliefs control our genetic activity, it gives us the power to maintain our health—regardless of what genes we have."

Bruce Lipton

Because I hold the belief that the body heals itself, doesn't imply that I believe Western, "fix me" medicine has no place. If I were in an accident and bleeding, with broken bones, I would welcome conventional medical diagnosis and treatment. I'm very thankful for the effective emergency treatment that I received after my hang glider crash, which was instrumental in saving my life. But it comes with a price.

Detoxifying your environment includes more than avoiding radiation, toxic cosmetics and cleaning products. It includes medications, which are all poisons, as they poison some normal pathway or function, in an attempt to lessen symptoms. They have their place in emergency situations, but are not in any way a "cure" or healthy long-term management strategy. Have you noticed how the prescriptions just seem to multiply? You start on one and soon you're taking five, as more problems keep cropping up. This is very good for the stockholders of the pharmaceutical companies, but it isn't the road to vibrant health.

Much of Western medical research concentrates on identifying "bad genes" or particular chemicals that predispose us to one disease or another. I'd like to take a moment to explain the difference between causation and correlation. Genes like BRCA1 and BRCA2 have been *associated* or *correlated* with a higher risk of breast cancer. But they don't **cause** it. Causation is seldom proven in medicine because so many diseases are the result of the interaction of many factors. It's much easier to find single things that can be shown to be associated or correlated statistically.

Worrying about having a particular gene, may be worse than having it! Remember how our thoughts affect our bodies at the highest level? Bruce Lipton's book, "The Biology of Belief" explains much more about the importance of environment and how it affects gene expression, if you would like to learn more about the science of epigenetics.

Your DNA may load the gun, but environment pulls the trigger. In other words, what we choose to eat, the toxins we take into our bodies and stress all have the potential to switch genes on or off. This is actually good news. We can switch off the "bad" genes and switch on the genes that are protective.

Having grown up in the Wild West, in a home where there were always loaded guns at hand, it's interesting to note that we didn't have a single incident or accident involving one of those guns. Nor did anyone we knew. Why? Because we were taught how to handle (and how not to handle) a loaded gun. We were taught discipline and self-control.

You knew this was coming. This is where I tell you that you must develop the discipline and self control to do what you know will contribute to your health and stop doing those things that you know you shouldn't. Not because I say so, but because they work against you.

Of course it will feel uncomfortable at times, when you make changes. That place of uncertainty is where you can begin to create your future; a brighter future of your own choosing, that may not only be different, but better than you ever imagined.

Cavett Robert defined character as "following through on a decision long after the excitement and emotion of the moment has passed'." Are you ready to start building character?

Write down what you are going to **do** today, that *you* know you should do, to start improving your health.

Write down what you are going to **stop** doing today that *you* know is detrimental to your health.

Make these changes for a whole week and you will have made a good start in turning your health around.

If you do this every week, adding one positive thing and eliminating one detrimental thing, while maintaining the changes you've already made, you will stay on the path of vibrant health.

Note: Nothing is 100%, so don't expect to follow your new program perfectly, all the time. And especially, don't beat yourself up when you don't. Feeling bad or guilty about not exercising or about eating that big slice of non-organic strawberry cheesecake, is worse for you than "cheating". If you're going to temporarily ditch your new habits for an hour, or a day, at least enjoy whatever you decide to do to the max! You will learn from your own experience what you can occasionally get away with and which things just aren't worth the consequences.

Chapter 8 - The Power of Belief

"Whatever the mind can conceive and bring itself to believe, it can achieve."

-Napoleon Hill-

If you're expecting me to tell you what to believe in order to become well and healthy, you still aren't getting it. Belief is a very powerful and necessary ingredient in your personal wellness recipe. And that is exactly why you will have to honestly assess what YOU believe.

Others can tell you what worked and didn't work for them. They can tell you of their faith in one religion or another. Only you and God, Supreme Being, The Infinite, Higher Power, Universe, Source...whatever name you choose, really know what you truly believe.

Will it help you to know what I believe? I doubt it. Except maybe for three things. These three things appear in the writings of every major religion I have studied and are close enough to absolute truth that they seem to create results whenever and by whomever they are applied.

First, we are immortal spiritual beings, having a physical experience - we are so much more than our bodies and minds. Why is this important to me? For me, it eliminates the fear of death. Fear causes us to put our attention on a perceived danger, making those things we fear happen. How can immortal spiritual beings die? The answer is in the question, they can't. It also puts life on earth into perspective. When I look at the big picture, what others think becomes way less important than what I KNOW. Learn to listen to your intuition, that part of you that KNOWS. Then, have the courage to BE who you really are!

Second, all things are possible to those who believe. Some think they have to see it to believe it, but I know that it's the other way around ... you have to believe it to see it. If you think you can or if you think you can't, either way you're right. To someone without faith, everything is a coincidence. To those who KNOW, life is a joyous journey, with help constantly available to let you know when a course correction is advisable. There are no failures, just some delays or changes in direction. If you know where you are now and where you want to go, plotting the course is fairly simple.

Third, unconditional love not only creates miracles, it is available to us at all times, if we stop pushing it away. Learning to give and accept love releases healing energy. Love opens your "eyes" so that you can see beyond the obvious. How often do we get upset and complain when something "goes wrong"? When someone doesn't act the way we want them to? When something doesn't happen the way we expected it to? If we were in a place of unconditional love, would we be upset about those things or people?

My prayer for you is that you experience this state of love, acceptance and faith that whatever happens, it is part of your journey, created by you, for your enlightenment. Whether or not you become physically well, you have a wonderful opportunity to become spiritually well and experience more joy in life than you have, thus far. Make the most of every minute, of every hour, of every day. Life is an adventure to be lived as fully as you can. Need I say more?

Appendix

A - Additional Reading

1. Bollinger, T. (2013), Cancer Step Outside the Box, Infinity 510(2) Partners

2. Campbell, C. T and Campbell 11, T. (2006), The China Study, BenBella Books, Inc.

3. Chopra, D. (1987), Creating Health, Houghton Mifflin Co.

4. Cousins, N. (1979), Anatomy of an Illness, WW Norton & Co, Inc.

5. Hay, L. L. (1984), You Can Heal Your Life, Hay House, Inc.

6. Hicks, E. and Hicks, J. (2004), Ask and It Is Given, Hay House, Inc.

7. Lipton, B. (2005), The Biology of Belief, Mountain of Love/Elite Books

8. McTaggart, L (2002), The Field, Harper Collins Publishing

9. McTaggart, L (2008), The Intention Experiment, Free Press Publishing

10. Morter, M. T. (1995), Dynamic Health, Morter Health System

11. Sarno, J. E. (1991), Healing Back Pain, Time Warner Book Group

12. Siegel, B. S. (1986), Love, Medicine and Miracles, Harper & Row

13. Trudeau, K. (2005), Natural Cures "They" Don't Want You To Know About, Alliance Publishing

14. Trudeau, K. (2006) More Natural "Cures" Revealed, Alliance Publishing Group

15. Wahls, T. (2014), Transcript of "Mitochondria, Health, and Vegetables", retrieved from: https://www.bulletproofexec.com/wp-content/uploads/2014/05/Transcript-120-Dr.-Terry-Wahls.pdf

16. Wahls, T. and Adamson, E. (2014), The Wahls Protocol: A Radical New Way to Treat All Chronic Autoimmune Conditions Using Paleo Principles, Avery Publishing

17. Weil, A. (1996), Spontaneous Healing, The Ballantine Publishing Group

B – Videos and Links

1. Carter, Al, ReboundAir Healthy Cell Concept (5 parts on YouTube), retrieved from: https://www.youtube.com/watch?v=rLMpWCou0l4

2. "The Knowing", Documentary (2016) with Bob Proctor, Les Brown, Janis Johnson, Bob Shontz, Mary Miller

3. Free online self improvement courses, retrieved from: http://www.scientology.org/courses.html

4. Holden, Lee, 7 Minutes of Magic (for Health), retrieved from: https://www.youtube.com/watch?v=cXfKWm2QBAE

5. How and why to do an elimination diet, retrieved from: http://www.precisionnutrition.com/elimination-diet

6. Holden, Lee, How to Use Simple QiGong to Transform Your Health and Longevity,

retrieved from:
https://www.youtube.com/watch?v=bnWspa
qJ5VY

7. Kinesiology Self Testing, retrieved from:
https://www.youtube.com/watch?v=gcXpDnT
mEjo

8. Pilates for Beginners, retrieved from:
https://www.youtube.com/watch?v=gcgbXDP
aFVw

9. The Pulse Test, retrieved from:;
http://soilandhealth.org/wp-
content/uploads/02/0201hyglibcat/020108.co
ca.pdf

10. Wahls, T., Minding Your Mitochondria,
retrieved from:
https://www.youtube.com/watch?v=KLjgBLw
H3Wc